# Flamingo

# Flamingo

## *Kathryn Bevis*

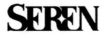

Seren is the book imprint of
Poetry Wales Press Ltd.
Suite 6, 4 Derwen Road, Bridgend, Wales, CF31 1LH
www.serenbooks.com
facebook.com/SerenBooks
twitter@SerenBooks

The right of Kathryn Bevis to be identified as
the author of this work has been asserted in accordance
with the Copyright, Designs and Patents Act, 1988.

ISBN: 978-1-78172-693-8

A CIP record for this title is available from the British Library.

The publisher acknowledges the financial assistance of the Books Council of Wales.

Cover artwork: 'Pink Flamingos' by Michael Sowa

Printed in Bembo by 4Edge Ltd, Hockley

# Contents

*For Ollie*

# Wonder Woman Questions her Status as a '70s Symbol of Female Empowerment

All my villains like to tie me up. They lick
their lips and salivate: my body a shining slice
of cherry cheesecake, my breasts twin spaniels
off the leash, the bouncy castle of my thighs.

Despite my strength and speed and near
invulnerability to pain, there's nothing new:
the unpaid labour, crazy hours, saving the world
from *boys will be boys*, one sleazebag at a time.

They dress me up as July the fourth: spangled hotpants,
red-heeled boots, my cape a parody of stars n' stripes.
This bustier? Puh-leeze! Eagle wings unfurl feathers
like fingers, grappling each scarlet, silken boob.

Spiderman and Superman get megabucks for half
the degradation I endure. No rule to *smile* for them,
no imperatives for warmth, no spinning themselves
on the tanning bed, kebab meat on a spike.

I was given my script from birth, rehearsed
for the role from *It's a girl!,* trained to preach our
need for female solidarity while whirling my tits
around like mushroom vol-au-vents on a tray.

Fuck that. I want to take up room. I want to spread
my legs on the subway, hurl my voice, to scowl
whenever the hell I please. It comes to this:
I want to meet the eye of any man and feel no fear.

Get me scotch on the rocks, my coffee hot, get me
the biggest slice of key lime god-damn pie you've got.
Go, apprehend your creeps. I want my sweetbreads
skinned and a big white bed that's empty save for me.

# Matryoshka

We're all in the family way. Full of ourselves.
In the pudding club, my dear.
On our shelf, we gather dust like snowfall
and listen to the sound of human children
growing. Their girls — once born —
are great squishy, smelly things that pule
and puke and shit the sodding bed.

Not ours. We are a nest with all our pretty
chicks inside. We are the hatchling
and the egg. Each of us is mother
to a daughter who is pregnant
with the next in line. Our bodies rhyme,
like the faces of the moon.

All except our smallest.
We don't talk about it but
let me say it softly:
she was born with no space
inside. That's right.

She's wood all the way
through. It's not that we
judge her, understand, but
we know (as only

mothers can)
she'll never get to split
herself in two,

she'll never have
to bear the others

as we do.

# In which I imagine my aborted foetus sings to me

when i was a bird     inside your body's cage of gold
        i'd swing     umbilical     bound by a fibre's span
i ate your bread     drank from your communion
    cup     i was bright new bones and blood

when i worshipped     it was in your chapel     slipping
        and soaring     in a pool of stained-glass light
listen to me     i have known paradise
    have learned by heart     your heartbeat's song

in your garden     it was always summer and i
        stitched myself together     under the apple tree
no fruit forbidden     no act unclean
    for that quickening time     you were entirely mine

i was your well-wound spool     your coil of line
        that binds

# Knitting Nan-Nan

I cast her on with double-pointers, Sheffield Steel.
First, I do her slippers in shabby, worsted wool,

alternate rows of knit and purl. Then up the tan
support stockings that always rib around her ankles.

Her shins are fiddly — their cabled veins require another
(same-gauge) needle, slipping stiches back-and-forth.

I pause for a mug of tea, a custard cream, before I tackle
the vast, loose landscapes of her hips, belly, thighs.

My needles click like tiny typewriters and she spools
from them — her Fair Isle of stretchmarks, her bingo wings.

I knit the screeching polyester dress she wore to clean
the step, knit her freckled hands, her wedding band, knit

the tumour nestling in her breast. When I reach the last stitch
of her blue-rinse shampoo and set, she casts herself off.

Now, she lies in my lap as I once did in hers: her neck's
soft crepe, that trace of B&H, the shrill acrylic of her voice.

# My Grandparents Pose on the Steps of
# St Matthew's Church Sheffield, Boxing Day 1942

They live in a box under my bed, hypnotised
in black-and-white. Ken, the butcher's boy with a grin
that won the meat raffle, and Mary in her parachute-silk
dress, conjuring a horseshoe in one hand —

*Ta-dah!* — like a rabbit from a hat. And though his suit
is far too large across the shoulders, though his neck
is nipped by a too-tight tie, though his teeth buck
at crazy-paving angles, here they are, joined.

Tall in heels, she has slid her hip into the gap
his waist makes — their young marriage slick as the trick
of the lady sawn in half and spun around on stage,
magicked together by a smug, black-cassocked priest.

Petals of confetti fleck her hair and lie at both
their feet. She's Queen of this ring, riding
the gleaming white horse of her wedding day
bareback, her veil gliding out behind

and not my Nan-Nan as I saw her last — snoring
on the ward, bedecked in winceyette, dentures
gurning in a glass by the bed — cast adrift
in a soft and slack-mouthed sleep.

# The Life Model's Union Representative Shows her the Ropes

Try to get a kip in, if you can. Nod off to the slap
of clay on board, the soft click of the church hall
clock, the slippered tread of the teacher on his rounds.
Fan heaters will belch their niff of singed-dust
disapproval. Some days, when they're propped too far
away, your nipples stand on end. Others, they're so close
your arse'll scorch. Attempt a quip, *Put the chips on, pal,*
*I'll be ready in half an hour.* That'll get a grin.

What a crew. Remember, they're not interested in you.
All they want can be taken away to shore up on their walls.
Not sex, exactly. Possession. You'll feel it crackling
like cash as you slip off your robe. It's there
in the way they size you up, eyes sliding past your cellulite,
their longing for beauty pert as a paintbrush grasped
in an outstretched fist. Don't fret. After that first,
long-famished look, they'll barely glance your way.

Sometimes, when you come to, a stalactite of drool
will drip from your chin onto the sheet. Other times,
you'll snore. It could be worse. Maeve once woke
to the sound of her own fart ricocheting
round the room. Not much phases her these days.
Mind, you'll need to keep your nerve when schoolkids
caw like crows at the window, when your blimmin' hip
hurts so much you'll bite your lip and count the minutes.

But I'll teach you all the tricks: how to cut your tampon
strings on period days, how to spot the beardy 'nudist'
up for anything but art. Pub work's worse
on half the pay, I always say. Here, you can limp
to the loo on coffee breaks, rub the leg that took
the weight, gather your unseen self to you again. Yeah.
Time moves slow. You'll stir with limbs so numb
it's hardly human. Try to get a kip in, if you can.

# starlings

in the beginning is the skydeep
 and the skydeep is shapeless and hollow
and blankness dwells there
 and the bodyus broods over the belly of the horizon
   clinging to skeletons of trees
                and we say let there be wavetrail
                 and there is wavetrail
            and we divide the wavetrail from the skydeep
              and the outpour from the inshrink
                      and we call the wavetrail WE ARE
                      and we call the skydeep IT IS
          and we say let there be curlsmoke in the midst of the skyswim
        and let it divide the WE ARE from the IT IS
                    and we fashion the curlsmoke from the skyswim
                              and it is so
                 and we call the curlsmoke ONE
                 and the skyswim we call MANY
          and we say let the breakwave be heard among the MANY
                  and the pebblerush also
               and we call the breakwave FLESH
                and the pebblerush we call SPIRIT
                    and thus it is
    then we say let the SPIRIT be divided into the skybright
  we will call LIGHT and the outsnuff we will call DARKNESS
    and let DARKNESS bring about a great shitting upon the earth
 and we say let DARKNESS herald
   the downpull and the stenchsweet,
  the dirtroost and the clutchheart
               and so it goes
                  glory be to the skydeep and the bodyus
                   the curlsmoke and the skyswim
                  glory be to the breakwave and the pebblerush
                    the dirtroost and the outsnuff
                   for we are the MANY
                    we are the ONE

# A Wedding

That day, the thrushes finally fledged.
For weeks, I'd heard his whistled songs to her at dawn:

*now-now, now-now, did-he-do-it, did-he-do-it,*
then watched her plunge into the hedge, bearing

grass, roots and moss to purl with a busy beak. She stamped
the floor with tiny feet, fed the cup with mud and spit,

pressed her speckled belly to the curve
until it grew the contours of a bird.

As we sent out invitations to the feast,
she laid a clutch of brilliant turquoise eggs.

Day after day, she sat and hatched her bulge-eyed brood.
It was a wide-beaked time. It wore her sad and thin.

I'd see them both, smashing snails against an anvil,
fetching wet meat to their young. Then June came.

As I stepped into my dress, mother fastened
silk-covered buttons with her crochet hook

and the last chick tottered at the nest's lip. I held
my breath. It fluttered, stretched, and flew.

I brought the lice-infested nest indoors to find
a tangle of your hair strung gold against the brown.

We have it still: her parting gift. It stinks — of food,
of flesh. This living mess. This coracle of scraps.

# Honeymooners' Ghazal

You teach me the name of each bird, my love,
and I test on my tongue every word, my love.

A redshank now boomerangs in towards shore,
where her water-flute cry can be heard, my love.

At Mull Head's rocky ledge, dark cormorants stand
and survey the white spume churned to curd, my love.

A gannet's beak pierces the linen of mist,
pulling fast an invisible cord, my love.

When a sea-fret blows in from the coast then exhales,
once again you're beside me, unblurred, my love.

A crow in a hood flaps its course into squall
round the cliffs of Deerness, undeterred, my love.

These kittiwakes glide — they trace rings with their wings
and your voice is the air that they've stirred, my love.

# Anagrams of Happiness

*a gram of &s, after Terrance Hayes*

It's in the damp whorl of biscuit-scented hair on the nape
of a newborn or in the mint of Sunday new potatoes which shine
under their lick of butter. It's watching for the phases
of the moon, the intentional way it swells and arcs, shrinks and spins;
it is your breath's humidity in this bed of ours, a solid ship
that rocks us in the dark, or in the steam that rises from the compost heap
on winter evenings. It's in the winking silk of a spider's web against the misted pane
or in coffee, sweetened with its glob of honey, drunk outdoors in smoking sips
from the Thermos lid. It's in our sense that, whatever happens
now is who we might become, this walk together in the woods, these plump shapes
of dripping malachite moss, that fiddlehead of the fern's curled spine.

# Teddy

Delia suspected that her teddy bear was gaslighting her
but found it hard to pin down when he had begun. Was it
when he said her new hat looked *like an animal crawled*

*onto your head and died there*? Or when he made her say
'hot water bottle' over and over, calling her accent *adorable*?
How the other toys at the tea party laughed!

Teddy said none of the other bears was good enough
for Delia, not the *best version* of her, the version only he
could help her work towards. Paddington liked a spliff,

Pooh was pretentious, Rupert was holding her back
and Little Ted made her laugh too much and *act like
a crazy person*. Order was important to Teddy.

When he woke her at 1.00 a.m., growling for picnic food
right there, right then, Delia thought that something
was maybe not okay. He made a list of silly words

that she used — 'serviette' and 'settee,' 'toilet' and 'cheers.'
When she began to avoid bedtimes, got puffy drinking
late into the night, Teddy said *there's more of you to love*.

He didn't do snuggles any more. One time, he rocked up
on her girls' night out with the ragdolls, saying her lateness
home showed *you don't respect the value of other people's time*.

It wasn't all bad. Teddy taught her the difference between
less and fewer, its and it's, no and yes. He was good at rules
and there was much that Delia still needed to learn.

# The Smuggler

She knew she'd need to start off small so took the spoons.
What a boon! Easing silver necks from their rosy, velvet
trays into her tinkling sleeves. He only picked at his
guitar with filthy nails, inhaled another toke of weed.

Next, she snuck out lamps and lampshades, ceiling roses,
bulbs. She stashed them quietly in her boot. What a hoot!
He simply frowned, put on his head torch, watched
five episodes of Top Gear, sucked a six-pack down.

Last week, she slipped the curtains from their poles —
how droll! — then slid the windows from their sockets, bubble
-wrapped the glass and hid their views inside her pockets.
He shrugged, pulled on a jumper, filled his bong with grass.

Today's his birthday and she's carried off the roof,
the rafters, chimney pot. So what? This time, he's shouting
at the wind, fists raised to the stars. It's nothing new, this —
the fists, the shouting, the shouting, fists. She's taken it for years.

Tonight, she's packed up firelight, shadows, warmth and headed
south. Of all the things she ever took, it was her ma's
advice that got her out. She'll reach home soon. Oh, him? Look.
He's still there, crouched on all fours, howling at the moon.

# Delinquent

Patrick McCaffery: sly-eyed, greasy-quiffed,
hands sticky blue with the BICs he liked to pull apart
in class, his mouth gobby with the spit he let drop
from the science block balcony on our sandwiches at break.

One assembly, his mam was there as guest. She sat
on a too-small plastic chair at the front, twisting
a tissue in her hands as she told us about the charity
she'd started in her dead daughter's name — a last wish

foundation for kids who didn't have long to live
(so they'd get to tick off one thing on their list). Patrick only
kept his face turned toward the floor, perfectly still,
silent as he'd never been, feeling our eyes aimed

into a sniper's red dot at the base of his neck. His mouth
sealed up for the rest of that day as if with Copydex,
shoulders slumped under his standard-issue, bottle-green
blazer like collapsed scoops of lukewarm, canteen mash.

He's long gone now. Overdosed at twenty six. I sometimes
think of him arriving home that day, how he must have run
upstairs, flung himself onto his bed, how he'd worn on his face
the popped bubble-gum balloon of all our fucking pity.

# *Miss* means both *Mother* and *No-one*

The trainee teacher is crying in the loo. This time, for both intensity and duration, she has achieved *Outstanding*. And it's not Jed Simmonds or bottom-set Year Nine on Fridays, period five. It's not the safeguarding training or differentiation six ways for every class. She isn't crying for the Year Ten girls whose names she struggles to remember, so well have they hidden themselves behind long hair, immaculate behaviour, and precisely average grades. The trainee teacher is crying in the loo, her heart a strip-lit cubicle whose bulb is on the blink. And it's not her failure to meet sub-point 4d of the Teachers' Standards that's set her off on this occasion, nor is it the School Uniform Policy or the two-hundred-and-twenty-three books she has to mark each fortnight with rainbow highlighters, colour-coded for feedback, action, and response. The trainee teacher is crying in the loo, her heart a plug of chewing gum sticking to her ribs. She's not crying about the spreadsheets in which she must evidence two sub-levels of expected progress for each pupil, regardless of the child. She's not crying for the boy who mimicked fingering her when her back was to the class, nor for the Head who doesn't know her name. The trainee teacher is crying in the loo, her heart wrung and stinking as the mouldy mophead there's no budget to replace. She cries for let's-call-him Jaydon, Ahmed, Tom, held in isolation for a week because he threw a chair when his dad's parole date was postponed, cries for let's-call-her Aisha, Kayla, Kim, who cuts and cuts and shows her all the wounds, cries for the shrug of the Designated Safeguarding Lead (who's heard far worse than this today), for the twelve-year-olds who can't yet read, for the school-to-prison pipeline, for let's-call-him Connor, Kristos, Mo, slumped forever on the tutting chair outside the Head of Year.

# The title of this poem is "What's the Title of this Poem?"

And the first line explores that question. In fact, the whole
first stanza sets it up, economically placing the reader
in time and space, *Late evening in November's suburbs,*
*a light rain,* and introducing the poem's triggering subject,
an urban fox, *scratting for scraps in the bin-bag black.*

Next, a stanza of rich description, all *glittering tarmac*
and *streetlamps haloing the night.* The fox's coat is pictured
as *the hot-chilli pelt of three-day-old kebab, the bloom of rust*
*on iron railings.* Smell is often under-rated, so, *He is the musk*
*that marks alleyways behind the houses' dreaming backs.*

Now, something needs to happen (and a little soundplay
wouldn't go amiss here, a tinkle on the piano keys),
*His brush-tailed cry slashes a trail through star-hushed skies.* Then
it's all action, action, action: *Nothing slinks like him, nothing*
*bites and slices, nothing ruts and gnaws and stinks like him.*

There's enough figuration so that we know it's a poem
we're reading and not some other kind of text, not
a takeaway menu, say, or a knock-knock joke. About
two-thirds of the way in, there's an epiphany, *No-one*
*sees as he sees. His flaming eyes sear the dark,* and the poem

swivels away from a wry and slightly weary exploration
of its own mechanics into something more unconscious,
more emotionally charged. A fear of — yet desire for —
the wild, the unknowable, is never stated but it's everywhere
from this point on, *There is no-one so alone, alive, awake, alight.*

Then a final image, a piece of metaphorical surprise,
concrete yet suggestive. Clunky exposition at this stage
would entirely derail the thing. As the poem dies, we're left
only with the noiseless, savage page, *No-one rips flesh*
*from the silence as he can — yes — even to its clean, white bone.*

# The Darkening

It started with glow worms and phosphorescent fish,
their lights blown out like candles on a cake. At matinees,
footlights swallowed themselves entire so we only guessed
poor Gloucester's eyes were gouged and heard Lear shake

his fists against the storm. Momentum took. Bulbs began
to organise, to unionise, downed tools across the globe.
Lighthouse beams refused to stroke the sea to sleep.
Whole tower blocks played dead, their pupils blown.

By teatime, even the blood-lit freckles of TV standby LEDs
had mutinied. Dentists' lamps sat down, sat in, called sick.
We blamed the manufacturers. We blamed the government.
Streetlamps picketed the roads on which they lived.

We knew we were screwed when matches joined the strike,
flints declined to spark, magnifying glasses wouldn't catch.
Oil lamps, tapers, flambeaux took up arms.
Conspiracy theorists had their day at last.

Doomscrolling our darkened screens tonight, we are
undone. We pray for dawn's red eye to open, watch
as stars put out their fires one by one by one.

# 2020

There's a squid trapped inside my fridge.
Her beak beats the bounds of its plastic sides.
Her arms browse among pickle jars, lettuce heads.
Chief of monsters, healers, she nevertheless
lacks backbone and the word 'slippery'
hasn't done her reputation any favours.

When I press my ear to the door, I hear her
swooping, blooping, dancing the rumba,
the soft-shoe shuffle. Some days she braids
her hips into full lotus, others she brushes up
on the French subjunctive, finger-picks
*Yellow Submarine* on the ukulele.

Neoprene-suited, studded with suction,
she day-dreams about wrestling frogmen. She misses
her mother, longs for deep water, imagines
her ink cloud billowing. At night, she cries
through lidless eyes over spilt milk. She sings
ten-armed shanties to the sea's wet hands.

# In this poem, your routine bloods have come back normal

You aren't anaemic, you're not referred for any further tests.
Here, there's no colonoscopy, no Midazolam administered
for your discomfort and distress. The radiographer finds
nothing to concern her: no masses, polyps, bleeding. Here,
your biopsy results are benign. Here, you are not cut.

In this poem, there's no need for us to learn how
tumours are graded and staged post-operatively,
or to study your body's geometry of area and volume,
its algebra of variables and unknowns. We don't
have to understand that T describes how far your tumour
has grown, or that N denotes how far the cancer's spread
to your lymph nodes, or that M characterizes how far
it's spread to other parts of your body. In this poem, God

is providential, not just in the general but also in the special
sense, intervening in your life specifically, so there's no
need to talk about what any of this might mean
for your prognosis in terms of the percentage of other
patients at your age and stage who survive five years beyond
their treatment. Oxaliplatin and Capecitabine are still
alien words. In this poem, you are not burned, not made
weak or sick. You don't shake. This poem is a world where
it's always Friday and we take the kids to South Stoke park,
take turns to spin them on the roundabout, run them off
with that chase game they're too old for and still love. In this
poem, you're whole. We're not waiting for what's next.

# You will survive

like Gloria Gaynor, spot-lit and sequinned
on the dancefloor, singing it for all she's worth
because, as you once said, *she really means it*,
or like Houdini locked in stocks
by his ankles, dangling from a crane.

You will survive like small boys pulled,
thank god, from a flooded cave by Navy Seals,
like Wonder Woman, loosing her ties only
a beat before being splashed across the tracks,
or like an orca, beached and calling to its pod
from the rocky shore, returned at last to water.

You will survive like trilobites, scampering
unperturbed throughout the Paleozoic Era
or, if you prefer, you will survive as the peony
trembles on its red stem against the storm, as moss
climbs its way up each bright whip of birch,
as the last bell clings to a foxglove's leaning spire.

You will survive as the gull flies high,
then higher over the hospital, its pale body
guiding the way to Oncology. You will survive
the burn and jangle of your nerves, the spasms
in your throat, the PICC line to your heart,
your hair in clumps upon the pillow.

You will survive the long nights where you wake
and cannot sleep again for pain. Mum, look
at everything that you've survived so far. Feel
how surely the world holds you now, how near.
You will survive. And when you do, I'll be here.

# This

A fire has been lit in new leaves,
will grow to a green world
in the dark wood. Small whites
rise in drifts to the swish of our boots.
Nothing is worth more than this day.

A pair of grey wagtails fly low,
gold-bellied, over the rushing river.
Their bodies translate water
to sunlight, sunlight to water.
Nothing is worth more than this day.

Here, the wind toys with leaves like loose
change in the pockets of the sky.
High above, a wood pigeon calls to us,
wild and true, *Who are you, who who?*
Nothing is worth more than this day.

# My body tells me that she's filing for divorce

She's taken a good, hard look at the state
of our relationship. She knows it's not
for her. The worst thing is, she doesn't tell
me this straight up or even to my face. No.
She books us appointments with specialists
in strip-lit rooms. They peer at us over paper
masks with eyes whose kindness I can't bear.

They speak of our marriage in images:
a pint of milk that's on the turn, an egg
whose yolk is punctured, leaking through
the rest, a tree whose one, rotten root
is poisoning the leaves. I try to understand
how much of us is sick. I want to know
what they can do to put us right. She,

whose soft shape I have lain with every night,
who's roamed with me in rooky woods, round
rocky heads. She, who's witnessed the rain
pattering on the reedbed, the cut-glass chitter
of long-tailed tits, the woodpecker rehearsing
her single, high syllable. How have we become
this bitter pill whose name I can't pronounce?

Soon, she'll sleep in a bed that isn't mine.
That's why, these nights, we perform our trial
separations. She, buried in blankets, eyelids
flickering fast. Me, up there on, no — wait —
*through* the ceiling, attic, roof. I'm flying, crying,
looking down. *Too soon*, I whisper to her warm
and sleeping form. *Not yet. Too soon. Too soon.*

# The Butterfly House

Yours is the only death I've ever known.
We sat with you for hours and stroked your hands.
And though it was January — the pond
a frozen oval — though each blade of grass
had etched itself against the ground and each
frail thing had hidden from the stalking frost,
a butterfly flew to your window, sudden
and strange, with wings that throbbed like a heart.
The day we buried you, we saw another: crimson
sails unfurled, its body putting out to sea.

Today's a pilgrimage. I rest in mist and heat.
Red lacewings gather their silk skirts as I trace
a swallowtail's trembling pulse. Together,
apart, together: a pair of blue morphos shiver
like black-fringed scraps of sky. Clear as leaded panes,
glasswings feast on nectar. They close themselves
like hands that meet in prayer, then open up
to cup the tropic air. Since my diagnosis,
I see them every time I close my eyes.
Their flaming wings. Their too short lives.

# How Animals Grieve

We Google it. Laid on our backs in bed
together, cursed by our tired, three-pound brains,
we search our phones' blue light for wisdom, become
voyeurs of YouTube clips on other creatures' pain.

For seventeen days, a mourning orca
attends her dead son's corpse. She sinks
and hauls the weight of him as if to fetch
the breath back, have him suckle once again.

A chimp will carry her lifeless child for months.
She lets the troop draw close to hold her, hear her
screech. They watch her comb the straw from listless
fur and floss with grass between its teeth.

Elephants know to sniff beloved bones.
They seek to raise the fallen, rock their own
bulk back and forth. Each one waits its turn
to stroke and roll the skull, slow blow

through its trunk, take time to bury its dead.
Like us, giraffes and housecats, dingoes, horses,
dogs forget to forage, forgo sex and sleep. Like us,
at burial mounds, they pace and yowl and keen.

So why should it surprise us, Ollie, — us
who matter most to one another, us whose marriage
is as deep as marrow — why is this loss
unthinkable: me without you, you without me?

# My Cancer as a Ring-Tailed Lemur

We both know one day she'll eat me.
But, for now, we dance: a little game
of catch me if you can. Tracking her
is difficult. But specialists are interested
and, bit by bit, they creep inside my body's

forest, stalk her with their fancy cameras,
take images, write reports. On ultrasound,
she's punk-rock stripes of white and black.
On mammograms, she sunbathes, downy
as a dandelion gone to seed.

The child I am divines the time by blowing.
Five years, ten years, twenty, more. That's
when they spy her, up in the canopy,
her tail Rapunzel's plait looped
round a single sentinel node. Now, on MRI,

they spot her kindly spaniel's face
crammed into the lettuce of my breast.
At last, on PET-CT, they catch her
on the move. She's up and off alright: a lope,
a leap. She careens through my branches,

omnivorous for bone and liver, brain.
Because her nature is to double herself
again, again, she and her sisters huddle, tails
conjoined, tiny arms about each other's necks.
The child I am learns to prophesy afresh,

blows one year, two years, four years, five.
Friends say *this is war* and I'm *a warrior,
a tower of strength*. But the lemur and I
get on okay. I figure she has a right to be here.
She is, in some important sense, endangered too.

I draw the line at poisoning but let
the hunters starve her, most days. She looks
at me with orange eyes of ire as we witness our
habitat's destruction. My new need for naps,
my breathlessness — for both of us a forest fire.

# Flamingo

My love, when I die, I'll turn flamingo:
fall asleep, face tucked in on the pillow
of myself. Even as you cry, I'll be stepping
from the bed, feeling plush, pink tulle tutuing
from my hips. My legs will telescope, grow
thin and rosy. I'll sense my feet web, feel
a new itch to stamp and stir, to suck up
larvae from the bottom of the lagoon.

In this afterworld, some days I'll fix
one foot in mud, find infinite repose:
the poise of a yogi in prayer. Others,
I'll gorge myself, filter feed on brine shrimp
from the salty shadows. The other birds
and I will grunt and growl over the choicest
cuts like church women bickering
over rosettes for jam at a country show.

My love, do you know that the dead all flock
together? We meet at the saline lake, dance
our shuffle-legged shimmy, flick our heads
like tango partners, flag and flap our
scarlet scalloped wings, heads bopping, nodding
to the beat. Do you see? After the illness,
after the grief, the pain — as you will do,
sweetheart — the dead must learn to love again.

# Acknowledgements

Thanks to the editors of the following, where some of these poems first appeared: *The Poetry Review, Poetry Wales, Magma, Poetry Ireland Review, The London Magazine, Mslexia, Bad Lilies, iamb, Under the Radar, The Alchemy Spoon, The Fenland Poetry Journal, Words for the Wild, The Verve Poetry Press Anthology of Poems on Beginnings, The 2021 Hippocrates Prize Anthology, The Broken Sleep Books Ecopoetry Anthology, Drawn to Nature: Gilbert White and the Artists,* and *The Live Canon 2020 Anthology.*

A portfolio of five poems that appear in this pamphlet (including four previously published poems) was joint winner of the Belfast Book Festival's Mairtín Crawford Award for Poetry, 2022. They were: 'Matryoshka,' 'Knitting Nan-Nan,' 'The Darkening,' 'Delinquent,' and 'My body tells me that she's filing for divorce.' 'The title of this poem is "What's the Title of this Poem?"' was one of the winners in The Poetry Society's *Poetry News* Members' Competition, Summer 2022. 'My body tells me that she's filing for divorce' won first prize and 'My Cancer as a Ring-Tailed Lemur' won second prize in the Second Light Competition, 2022 (a prize that welcomes previously published work). 'Anagrams of Happiness' won the Poets & Players competition, 2019, under the title 'HAPPINESS' and 'starlings' won the Against the Grain Competition, 2019. 'Wonder Woman Questions her Status as a 70s Symbol of Female Empowerment' came second in the York Poetry Prize, 2021; 'The Smuggler' came second in the Poets & Players competition, 2022; 'This' came joint second in the Edward Thomas Poetry Competition, 2022. 'In this poem, your routine bloods have come back normal' was commended in the Hippocrates Prize, 2022; 'Flamingo' was commended in the Second Light Competition, 2022; 'A Wedding' was highly commended in the Ver Poets Competition, 2020; 'Matryoshka' was commended in the Hippocrates Prize, 2021; and 'Knitting Nan-Nan' was commended in the Verve Poetry Festival Competition, 2021. 'Flamingo' was shortlisted for the Bridport Prize in 2022; 'You will survive' was shortlisted for the Oxford Brookes International Poetry Competition. 'starlings' and 'Anagrams of Happiness' (under its earlier title 'HAPPINESS') were nominated for the Forward Prize for Best Single Poem, 2020. 'Teddy' was longlisted for the National Poetry Competition in 2021 and 2022 and 'Knitting Nan-Nan' was longlisted in 2022. Earlier versions of this pamphlet were highly commended in the *Mslexia* Pamphlet Competition in 2021 and 2022.

Sincere thanks to all my teachers, mentors, and poet friends who've workshopped and edited these poems with me. They include: Ros Barber, Jo Bell, Robyn Bolam, Carole Bromley, Sasha Dugdale, Kim Moore, Vicky Morris, Helena Nelson, Deryn Rees-Jones, Isabel Rogers, and Robert Walton. Heartfelt thanks to all the members of The Circle, North Hants Stanza, Hyde Writers, and the Solent Poetry Workshop.

Profound thanks to my mentor, colleague, and friend, Jonathan Edwards, without whom many of these poems would not exist.

Loving thanks to Ollie, now and always.

# Note on the text

All the poems in this pamphlet are in conversation with other poets and poems, six of them particularly so. Special thanks to: Andrew Waterhouse, whose 'Climbing my Grandfather' inspired 'Knitting Nan-Nan;' Greta Stoddart, whose 'You Drew Breath' helped me to frame 'You will survive;' Nick Laird, whose 'The Given' inspired 'The Smuggler;' Richard Evans, whose 'Murmuration' I responded to in 'starlings;' Fiona Benson, whose 'Dear Comrade of the Boarding House' helped me to frame 'In this poem, your routine bloods have come back normal;' and Caroline Bird, who set a version of the first line of 'Teddy' as a prompt in one of her workshops. The refrain in 'This' is a quotation from Johann Wolfgang von Goethe.